CONTENTS

KETTLEBELL FOR THE JIU-JITSU ATHLETE (SERIES TWO)

Mechanics, Protocols, Training Integration, and Training Periodization for the Athlete

Okonta kosi

INTRODUCTION

Hey Jiu-Jitsu lovers!

I know that you immensely loved the part one of this book, even as I loved writing every bit of writing it. In this new book, I delve deeper into more details of Kettlebell for the Jiu-Jitsu Athlete. These include the minute details about the Mechanics of Kettlebell along with its various Protocols that you will need to know in order to become a master within. Then, it will proceed to discuss the Training Integration and Periodization before talking about how you can train your energy system. You will be introduced to the concept of Tabata and this will aid you in the journey towards Jiu-Jitsu perfection.

Remember that you are going to be groomed in building your endurance levels at the end of this.

CHAPTER 1

KETTLEBELL MECHANICS AND PROTOCOLS

The world of kettle bell training is exceedingly large and often overwhelming with the many techniques and modifications, which are often introduced in the sport and as part of the Brazilian Jiu Jitsu training regimen for individual fighters. However, if you choose to pay more attention to a few solid basics and work really deeply and hard on them, you can kick off your journey towards building wonderful flows in your program and career in Brazilian Jiu Jitsu.

For example, you could decide to skip out on the sets and reps and focus more attention on the grace and elegance of your kettle bell skills. You can decide to lose yourself to the flow, working on several new transitions and progressions at a slow, yet steady pace. You can decide to move through each of these drills smoothly or you can decide to perform them slowly or quickly. The important fact to note is that whatever way you choose to approach this from, you are in charge of how you progress in developing your skill. Basically, you are in control.

Deciding which kettle bell regimens to focus more attention on is often considered a herculean task due to the many varied forms or techniques, which are available in kettle bell for Brazilian Jiu Jitsu. As a result of the dilemma which is often faced in the process of deciding which techniques to focus on, I decided to include some of my favorites in this book to help you get started.

1. The Kettlebell Rocking Chair: The first is a movement found in a lot of different Brazilian Jiu Jitsu techniques and transitions. It is usually performed using body weight only and often with the help of a kettle bell. This technique is efficient for improving excellent movement for hip/ knee mobility and for helping to build core strength. By including a kettle bell and a press, you are incorporating multiple muscles at the same time, increasing the possibilities of efficiency. This way, you will be working on your upper chest, biceps, triceps, shoulders and your core simultaneously. By the time you are done with this technique, you would be as fit as a ninja.

2. Deck Squats: These are like squats on but with extra, extra benefits like you are on steroids. By rolling from your back all the way to your feet, you incorporate a lot of different muscles; particularly, your core. There is a lot of getting up off your back to your feet in both MMA and Brazilian Jiu Jitsu so this one contributes tremendously to your general workflow and fitness for the mat.

3. Corner to Corner Rows: In Brazilian Jiu Jitsu, it is not uncommon that we do a lot of pulling from this position. So, it is important to incorporate a lot of different row variations in your work outs in order to get your body in the shape and form for when you would need to pull these moves during a sparring contest.

4. The Fighters Figure 8: This was also one of the first exercises developed when embarking on the Kettle jitsu journey. The idea is to incorporate punching as much as you can in your work out regime in order for you to get your arms in the shape and form for moving and maneuvering during a sparring contest. This one mimics the punching movement of a hooking type punch. It also addresses pivoting and torque. The effect of this can be felt on the upper part of your body and in your core simultaneously.

It is important to keep this in mind, before getting to the main work out, it is important to warm up first. The best way to go about this warm up is to get in plenty of body weight first. Then, the next step would be to practice each individual kettle bell exercise for 30 seconds with 10 seconds of rest in between. Once you drill each exercise for several rounds, then you can wrap it up with the final kettle bell pyramid.

CHAPTER 2

KETTLE BELL TRAINING INTEGRATION

One thing to take note of is the reality that you can definitely build strength with any form or range of added resistance from Dumb bells, Barbells or Power bags. However, Kettle bells do have one major distinguishing factor of advantage over most of the other pieces of the equipment and this factor or feature is the handle. The handle of the kettle bell is crafted in such a way that it is perfect for holding the weight of the instrument in several different positions.

An example, during the Kettle bell Press, the ball of the kettle bell lies against the forearm, offering a very comfortable position for the wrist which helps in the pressing of much larger weight. During the squat, the Kettle bell can be placed in the rack position and by nicely resting it against the upper arm and forearm, you can enable much larger weight to be held against the body.

These incredible instruments called kettle bells offer a nearly unprecedented amount of variety to train the shoulder girdle. Also, other than gymnastic rings which often require far more specialized training and strength, using kettle bells allows you the opportunity to train the shoulders through any anger and with any speed you can imagine. As a result of this, if your aim is to choose what the kettle bell does best, it is better to settle for the single-handed, cyclic in nature and the kettle bells that offer an ability to train the shoulder through large ranges of motion.

It is also important to note that large muscles are not necessarily the same as strength. To become strong enough, especially for the sport or during a specific lift maneuver, it is important to become efficient at the movement involved in that life maneuver. Efficiency of movement implies recruiting more motor units which, in turn, will help to kick start more muscle fibers to land greater contractile impact on the strength quotient. With constant practice, you can learn to educate your body to recruit the maximum amount of motor units to engage during each life and through this maneuver, you can improve and increase your strength.

Indeed, when many people commence their journey down the path of resistance training, also referred to as lifting weights, it is this efficiency of movement or motor unit recruitment that gives the impression of gaining muscle. The amateur weight lifter gets more skillful at lifting weights overtime and this helps to improve the strength of that individual much more than their muscle development. However, there surely comes a time when efficiency and motor recruitment are maxed out and additional muscle mass becomes the only way to improve and increase or further develop your strength.

SPINAL ALIGNMENT MECHANICS

When preparing for your sparring bouts in Brazilian Jiu Jitsu, it is important to take your kettle bell very seriously as they contribute greatly to the functionality and response of your spinal framework. To be in top form for your bout, you need to be free of any form of back pain and resistance training is especially helpful for eliminating back pain. It is very important to strengthen the body and increase anaerobic fitness in order to get into form for the sparring bout and this is a very wonderful way of achieving this. Resistance training can be performed in several forms ranging from bodyweight exercises, barbells, dumb bells, cables, machines, resistance bands, and kettle bells. The kettle bell is considered one of the more effective instruments to use for resistance training especially as a Brazilian Jiu Jitsu fighter. The kettle bell is a round, cast iron weight with a single handle – visualize a cannonball with a u-shaped handle. Kettle bells are manufactured in a wide range of weights for everyone from beginners to competitive strength athletes to the suitable weight classes for Brazilian Jiu Jitsu fighters.

Properly structured and functional kettle bell training increases aerobic and anaerobic fitness by developing the cardiovascular and musculoskeletal systems. Kettle bell training supplies a full body work out – the swinging of the instrument requires the movement of the entire body – by strengthening, toning, and helping the body to move bilaterally. It conditions all the major muscle groups to work together in order to ensure that the spine and back are properly conditioned for the performance ahead.

Kettle bell exercises strengthen the entire body, especially the spinal muscles for the back and the waist. They also contribute to the general functioning of your lifts during the fight. The shape of the kettle bell positions it as a versatile too for building strength and allows for a wide variety of exercises. Fundamental kettle bell exercises range from swings, to anchor squats, cleans, high pulls and push presses. All functional kettle bell exercises are combination exercises, meaning they force several major muscle groups to work together, functioning synergistically to bring about balance in the spinal muscles. Every single kettle bell exercise involves the spinal muscles and the core muscles.

The spinal muscles and the core muscles are often within the context of primary muscles involved in the process of the lift or functioning as auxiliary muscles in the process of the lift. Also, in all kettle bell exercises, the spinal and core muscles function in synergy to ensure stabilization in the body. As a result of this combination (always being involved in the movement, as well as always stabilizing the body), kettle bell exercises function for the training of the spinal muscles and helps to build power and stability in the spine, pelvis, hips and abdominal muscles. This is why it is important to take this exercise seriously for Spinal Alignment Mechanics.

Another thing to take note of is the fact that Kettle bell training is executed with large functional movements, high repetitions, perfect technique, momentum, and short rest periods between sets. As a result of this, the large functional movements ensure the entire body works in synergy. These types of movements simultaneously contribute to the strengthening of multiple muscles groups including the smaller supporting structures which are often inhibited or housed by the stronger muscles. This is different from a vast range of other of strengthening exercises that isolate specific muscles; kettle bell training relies on full body movements to lift the weight.

Also, in order to deliver maximum benefit and ensure injury prevention, it is very crucial to execute all kettle bell exercises with perfect technique. This point cannot be overemphasized, especially for Brazilian Jiu Jitsu fighters. It is important to work with a knowledgeable kettle bell instructor in order to learn proper technique for all exercises. Ensure that the trainer demonstrates as they teach, and supervise you during all phases of your training. Perfect your technique before increasing intensity and weight. It is important to note that for people who have gotten used to the process, this disclaimer is not necessary.

However, everyone (both amateur and pro) should understand that functional kettle bells training is a valuable tool in the advanced phases of preparing for a sparring bout and for injury rehabilitation and prevention, but it is not for everyone. If any kettle bell exercise elicits any discomfiting symptoms or doesn't quite feel right, then it is important to forego the exercises and focus on something else that functions better. Still, it is important for me to mention that kettle bell is the best form for people who hope to build strength for Brazilian Jiu Jitsu. If you enjoy kettle bell training and it feels right for you, then learn the exercises and perform them correctly and consistently to strengthen your spinal muscles and increase your health, fitness, and functionality.

CORE ACTIVATION

Kettle bells are very great for core activation – that is for getting your inner strength maximized for lifts and maneuvers during fights – and there are different processes for getting your core activated. Here, I have outlined the process of one of the more popular ways. This technique is referred to as the goblet squat.

To get started, get a kettle bell sitting between your feet hinge down and grab the bell by the handle, safely stand up and explosively lift the bell to your chest and jump your hands to the horns of the bell. The bell should be about 6" from your chest with your elbows forward and close to the bell.

While holding this position you can locate great trunk positioning by reaching your scapulae around your rib cage with the aim of activating your serratus anterior. Take a long breath out, to depress the ribs, and find a posterior tilt around the pelvis. This is the position you will maintain throughout the squats.

Inhale and bend at the hips and knees as low as your body can safely go without lifting your heels or toes off the floor. Most people define a good squat as hips below the knees, but when focusing on core alignment you should only squat as low as you can while maintaining proper positioning of the ribs, spine and hips. As you improve your core tension and mobility you will eventually reach a rock bottom squat.

Pause at the bottom of the squat to make sure you aren't bouncing and losing your core tension. You can use a mirror to the side to make sure your pelvis remains in posterior tilt. If you lose balance at the bottom, try holding the weight further away to counter any ankle tightness.

Brace the core and extend the knees and hips to return to the top of the movement. Make sure your toes, balls of the feet, and heels are all pushing through the floor on the way up. You should finish with hips still in posterior tilt and core braced.

HIP RECRUITMENT

Taking a cursory look at the foundational and fundamental structure of the hips is a viable way of determining how to go about hip recruitment. There are about six muscles that form a group and whose structure you can fairly place in comparison beside the rotator cuff muscles of the shoulder. In order to get more information on this, I'll suggest you read some more on the subject and consider a few visual aids to help form an understanding of the structure and pattern of the hips.

Combined with the ligaments, these muscles help the hip achieve a balanced sense of stability and positioning. From that point on, there are layers of muscles which allow the femur – often referred to as thigh bone – to move in any direction the body deems fit. Most of the hip muscles do different things including bringing the hip forward, rotating it inwards, moving it backwards and engaging in external rotation. Rather than focus on what each individual muscle can accomplish on its own, it is advisable to create a feeling of balanced strength and mobility throughout the range of motion of the hip. When you accomplish this, everything seems to work and feel much better than before and this gets you geared for the Brazilian Jiu Jitsu sparring bout.

Terrible hip extension is often associated with tight hip flexor muscles which are located at the front of the leg and stretch when you attempt to move your leg backwards behind you. To add to this tightness, a number of your hip flexor muscles are short and broad and these kinds of muscles are mostly difficult to stretch. The hip flexor muscles also tend to be hard for people who isolate for stretching or active movements which often require flexibility. In addition to that, there is the adductors and the abductors which function variedly for men and women but also functions extensively in the role of the mobility of your hip.

CHAPTER 3

TRAINING THE ENERGY SYSTEM

When it comes to preparing for a sparring bout in Brazilian Jiu Jitsu competitions, the process of doing the right strength and conditioning work outs can be very challenging for both amateurs and pros. The Brazilian Jiu Jitsu fighter must be prepared to put in varied amounts of effort at all times that he is training. A common example: sometimes, a fighter could be working towards getting a takedown which typically requires a great deal of effort and energy followed by a 20-30 seconds submission attempt, only for you to end up completely gassed. You could get swept off your feet, routed and end up on your back, on the defensive and fighting hard to survive the attempts of your opponent to submit you.

The intricate process of training your energy system will help you to learn how to tap into the different energy systems that the body uses for functionality. The problem or challenge many competitors face is that they are not familiar with expending diverse types of energy and working through different paces, and this makes it easy for them to gas out too early, too frequently. Many times, Brazilian Jiu Jitsu athletes harbor the notion that the only thing they need to be good at the sport is good cardio, and subsequently, they put in so much time running to benefit their Brazilian Jiu Jitsu. It is important to point out that this isn't out of line to do, however, the reality is that you can control the pace from running on a treadmill. You can speed up and slow down whenever you need to. However, in the actual competitive sport, your actions are all in reaction to the pace of your opponent. Either you are the one setting the pace and working hard to stay ahead, or you are the one fighting for your life and on the defensive, constantly at the mercy of your opponent and trying to match their pace. Whichever way it happens, your pace is often determined by the other person – unlike on the treadmill. Also, it is important to keep in mind the fact that when you roll, you are basically doing cardio and lifting weights simultaneously. No matter how good your technique is when you are framing in side control to escape or cranking on the arm for a submission, your opponent is resisting. In order to ensure you are in top form for a competitive bout, it is imperative to understand what energy systems are being utilized and what they are being utilized for.

In the sport of Brazilian Jiu Jitsu, the major energy systems that are put to use are the ATP system, the anaerobic system and the aerobic system. Before we proceed, let us consider the ATP system. Also referred to as Adenosine Triphosphate, ATP is a nucleotide which encapsulates a large amount of chemical energy which is stored in its high energy phosphate bonds. This nucleotide releases energy when it is broken down into Adenosine Diphosphate or ADP. The energy is often implemented in various metabolic processes. It is for this reason that the ATP is considered as the most universal energy currency for metabolism. This system distributes maximal energy outputs for a short duration in the absence of oxygen which usually lasts for about 10 seconds. Some examples of this energy system in action are shooting a takedown or throw and lifting heavy weights during exercise or during a sparring bout.

The second one; the anaerobic system simply refers to the absence of oxygen. This energy system consists of almost maximal energy outputs over a longer sustained period where oxygen demand accelerates higher than oxygen supply. This process often lasts within 2 minutes thereabouts. A few examples of this are submission attempts during a sparring bout and sprinting.

The last and more important energy system applied for Brazilian Jiu Jitsu sparring bouts is the aerobic system which involves the use of oxygen. The process of the system produces the largest amounts of energy but at the lowest intensity. This energy production can be held for extended periods of time provided breathing is able to supply sufficient oxygen to the lungs. Examples of this are transitioning through more than one positions, defending or holding a position, distance running and swimming.

The bottom line is that every Brazilian Jiu Jitsu fighter needs to know what energy system functions better for them in order to learn how to train that energy system and become proficient in the handling of that energy system while delivering a strike during a sparring bout or drilling or competitive bout. In this chapter, we will dive in and consider some other equally important aspects to the process of training the energy systems. We would identify certain energy systems and expand on how to train them to benefit the Brazilian Jiu Jitsu fighter for both sparring bouts and drilling exercises.

TABATA: THE ULTIMATE CONDITIONING METHOD

The concept of Tabata was propounded by Izumi Tabata who had been publishing research on the aerobic and anaerobic systems before his seminal work. He achieved most of his work by putting people through many different sprinting-type simulations in order to determine how and when the different energy systems of the body were used. ATP, the most important molecule used for energy production, is manufactured by both aerobic and anaerobic processes (in different ways). Tabata aimed to find a training program that would be the most efficient in improving this synthesis. As a result of his search, Tabata, in the early 1990s, he teamed up with Irisawa Koichi, the coach of the Japanese speed skating team, who had recently developed a protocol of short maximum bursts of sprints followed by short periods of rest. The program appeared to sustain and enhance peak performance in elite speed skating athletes, so Tabata wanted to test the protocol with athletes at different levels.

The initial Tabata Work out paper from 1996 evaluated two groups of amateur athletic males in their mid-twenties:

- The first group pedaled on an ergometer for sixty minutes at moderate intensity (70% of VO2 max). Similar to a long jogging session.

- The second group pedaled for 20 seconds, followed by 10 seconds of rest, for 4 minutes (completing 7 to 8 sets total) at maximal effort. The key phrase is maximal effort, as each interval was expected to be a sprint. If athletes could not keep up the speed requirements, they were stopped at 7 sets.

Tabata and his team conducted their research on two groups of varied athletes. The first group trained at a moderate intensity level while the second group engaged in training at a high-intensity level. The moderate intensity group worked out five days a week for a total of six weeks; each work out lasted one hour. The high-intensity group worked out four days a week for six weeks; each work out lasted four minutes and 20 seconds (with 10 seconds of rest in between each set).

The results; Group 1 had increased their aerobic system (cardio-vascular), but showed little or no results for their anaerobic system (muscle). Group 2 showed much more increase in their aerobic system than Group 1, and increased their anaerobic system by 28 percent. In the long run, the conclusion becomes that high-intensity interval training has more impact on both the aerobic and anaerobic systems.

Each exercise in a given Tabata work out lasts only four minutes, but it's likely to be one of the longest four minutes you've ever endured. The structure of the program is as follows:

- Work out hard for 20 seconds
- Rest for 10 seconds
- Complete 8 rounds

The aim is for the participating individual to push his body as hard as possible for straight 20 seconds and then take a 10-second break to rest. This is one set and you are required to complete eight sets of each exercise. You can do pretty much any exercise you wish. You can do squats, push-ups, burpees or any other exercise that works your large muscle groups. Kettle bell exercises work great, too.

An example of a Tabata work out looks like this:

- Push-ups (4 minutes)
- Bodyweight Squats (4 minutes)
- Burpees (4 minutes)
- Mountain Climbers (4 minutes)

Start with push-ups and perform them for about 20 seconds with a high-intensity. Rest for 10 seconds, and then go back to doing push-ups for 20 seconds. Once you complete eight sets of push-ups, rest for one minute. Next, move on to squats and repeat the sequence of 20 seconds on, 10 seconds off. Once you finish eight sets of squats, rest for one minute, and then do burpees. After burpees, finish the work out with mountain climbers. Tabata is great to get a quick work out in if you're short on time, you need to switch up your routine, or you want enhance your endurance and speed levels or limits. Switch up your work out or fitness routine if you want to break through with your fitness for your Brazilian Jiu Jitsu competitions.

METABOLIC CONDITIONING: EMOTM

Metabolic Conditioning work outs involve the use of exercises that burn lots of calories during your work out and help to keep the body burning calories even after your work out has come to an end. These kinds of work outs usually involve the entire body, short periods of rest in between and are meant to push the limits of your body with the aim of building strength and endurance while getting toned. The work outs under the Metabolic Conditioning are considered to be some of the toughest and most challenging exercise plans known to Brazilian Jiu Jitsu fighters on the planet. This means you will get the opportunity to improve your overall conditioning at a faster rate compared to your regular work out routines.

The metabolic circuits consist of power training, plyometrics, strength and conditioning, cardio, muscular endurance and core development. These metabolic circuits will help you improve your overall fitness – using your Bodyweight, Kettle bells, Dumb bells, Barbells, Medicine Balls, Stability Balls, Resistance Bands, Sandbags and other fitness equipment to jack up your metabolism, burn body fat and improve your overall work capacity.

Metabolic conditioning is not necessarily new on the work out scene and has been promoted by strength coaches for several years coming. With the explosion in popularity of MMA and Brazilian Jiu Jitsu, metabolic conditioning work out techniques and fitness routines have found their way onto the mainstream fitness landscape and are now being fully utilized by competitive athletes, hardcore fitness enthusiasts, and recreational work out practitioners alike. Metabolic conditioning is simply moderately resisted interval training using some combination of multiple joint body weight, suspension trainer, kettle bell, barbell, dumb bell, medicine ball, sand bag, sled, prowler and resistance band exercises. For those interested in or looking to get or remain strong and physically jacked, metabolic conditioning allows us to get all the heart healthy conditioning and fat loss benefits from engaging in traditional cardio and interval training, but without all of the drawbacks such as muscle loss, impeded recovery, boredom, and a substantial time commitment.

One of my favorite forms of metabolic conditioning is complexes. Complexes are basically defined as the performing of a series of multiple joint exercises, "strung together one after another with no rest, using the same resistance and the same number of reps on each exercise." One of my favorites – and most grueling – complexes involves performing 10 exercises: 8 using a single kettle bell, for a total of 200 reps. This complex will obviously enhance your level of conditioning, but it will also improve your power endurance and, by using offset or asymmetrical loading, you'll get an incredible core work out as well.

If you are going to use this exercise as a stand-alone conditioning work out on the days you do not strength train, I'd suggest modifying things a bit: instead of doing 10 reps of each exercise, cut it down to 5 reps. This brings the rep total to 100. Rest 2-3 minutes between complex circuits and perform 4-6 total complexes.

A lot of people are already familiar with the kettlebell swing by now. But it is important to note that by incorporating a few additional moves and one more kettlebell, you can get a fantastic work out benefit that can help fasten the process of building your muscle and setting your metabolism on fire.

This conditioning work out is a high-intensity, interval-based work out characterized by short periods of all-out effort followed by periods of rest. Over time, the capacity for work will increase, and this implies that you will have the ability to accomplish more work within a shorter time schedule. You'll notice that there is no prescribed number of reps for this work out – you should simply aim to complete more reps in the same amount of time or add more weight as you progress and your conditioning improves. This routine helps improve the lifts and rises and the maneuvers of your Brazilian Jiu Jitsu.

These all-out efforts followed by rest are more effective and burn more fat than a steady-state endurance training session because they trigger excess post-exercise oxygen consumption, or EPOC, more commonly known as the afterburn. This afterburn effect is the reason why intense exercise helps burn more fat and calories that steady-state work outs and produces a metabolism boost for up to 48 hours after you're done training. Your barbells and dumb bells are effective. The kettle bell is just an additional tool for your ability to burn fat and it breaks up the monotony of your more vanilla routine. The exercise list of the work out routines for Brazilian Jiu Jitsu and Grapplers includes the following;

1. DB Clean and Press

2. Burpee Kick Thrust

3. Alternating Knee Hip Thrusts

4. Rotating Burpees

5. Goblet Lunge

6. Bunny Hop Sprawls

7. Inverted Rows

8. Rolling Burpees

9. Sandbag Shouldering Side to Side Cleans

10. Burpee Thrusters Speed

CHAPTER 4

KETTLE BELL TRAINING PERIODIZATION FOR BRAZILIAN JIU JITSU

In order for your training with kettle bell to be effective, it needs to be consistent. In order for the body to get used to the routine and begin to exhibit the results from that training regimen, it is important to put it in consistent and constant practice.

Knowing when you should be resting and when you should be performing your kettlebell workouts will make a huge difference to the results you achieve along with minimalizing injury potential. We achieve results when we exercise by forcing our incredibly adaptive body to perform movements out of our comfort zone. As we push ourselves our body realizes that we are demanding something from it that it is not totally efficient at.

We are using more energy than usual, stretching soft tissue more than usual and using more motor neurons than usual. Just like every action in life we either move away from Pain or towards pleasure. Once the body experiences discomfort through exercise it then starts to adapt in order to prepare for future similar stimuli.

In other words, it thinks "Wow that workout was tough, I will need to make some changes to make it easier next time". It is during this ADAPTATION phase that all the good stuff happens. You lay down more muscle fibers, the energy system improves and

Kosi Okonta

soft tissue becomes more pliable.

THE 12-WEEK TRAINING PROGRAM

Once you understand the Adaptation Phase or Super- Compensation phase, you realize that rest between sessions is vital for recovery. Without rest our body cannot adapt and therefore we cannot improve. Now for the shocking part, depending on what type of training you are doing you may only need to exercise every 5 days over a course of 12 weeks. There are a few factors that determine how many days rest you require.

THE 8-WEEK OUT TRAINING PROGRAM

If you are working out to a high intensity and the overload on your system is great then the ability to rejuvenate and restore homeostasis will take longer. For example, multiple sets of heavy swings or deadlifts will take longer to recover from than a set of overhead presses because heavy swings and deadlifts use 100's of muscles at a time.

As you progress deeper into your workouts and start to lay down more muscle you will require more time to repair and restructure your system. This usually expands over a period of 8 weeks and extensively covers everything from kettle bells to cardio and rolling drills.

Conclusion

I really hope you enjoyed this ride. On a personal level, I wish you have a unique journey towards reaching the top of your game. There are many obstacles that will prove to be very difficult to scale through, but I want you to always remember that you have it within you to overcome! To aid you, I will drop some positive affirmations that you can learn and recite while in the course of your workouts. Over the course of time, they would definitely aid you in building your self-confidence.

- I deserve every good gift I get
- I do not wait to get motivated by others, I motivate myself
- I am the one responsible for my success
- I depend on myself to succeed
- The success of my life is dependent on me
- There is more to me than this
- I can be more, I can do more
- I work towards achieving my goals
- I work smart
- In the face of challenges, I am calm
- I love doing the right things
- I do all it takes to achieve my goals
- My goals are smart and achievable

- I am an intelligent goal getter
- I am not just a dreamer, I am an achiever
- I am empowered to achieve my goals
- I do not allow past experiences kill my zeal
- I do not make the same mistake twice
- I have the ability to concentrate for a long period of time
- I am disciplined enough to stick with my decisions
- I make decisions that make my goals achievable
- I get what I need to do done within the time frame
- I set targets and hit them
- I am conscious of all the potentials in me
- I achieve all on my to-do list.
- I am not a quitter, no matter how difficult the task is I will not quit
- I am proactive and productive
- My attention is not divided
- I am free from all distractions
- My eyes are set on the prize
- My abilities are constantly developing
- I easily focus on important things
- I have high level of focus

- I am super optimistic to do this.
- I make progress because I try.
- Trying this is the only way they can see how good I am at this.
- If I don't try, I'll never know if I can or not

- I choose to remain positive.
- I release positive vibes only

- If they think I can do this, who am I to think I can't.
- If God believes in my abilities and intelligence, I believe him
- I am capable of greatness.
- I will do this excellent without complaint.
- I use my resilience to press forward and achieve my goals.
- I embrace this feeling and turn it to fuel for great things.
- I will remember today for good, so let's go make this day memorable!
- I am nearing my dreams by doing this, so I will do it.
- I have intellectually outstanding and resilient to achieve do this task.
- This is progress masked as fear
- I unmask fear to reveal my strength and confidence.
- I possess the strength of character to achieve all my dreams.
- My dreams are not lofty, they are mine to achieve and surpass.
- Who will do this? Me! Me! Me!.
- I am a disciplined person.
- I have self-control.
- I am in charge of my emotions.
- I am in charge of my destiny.
- I am in charge of this light inside me.
- I let my light shine for the world to see.
- Fear can't take charge of a life I own.
- I take the wheels of my destiny off the hands of fear.
- This fear is unreal

•   Who I am is the realest thing here.